Weight Loss the Agile Way

ELENA FEDOROVA

Disclaimer:

This book provides insights into the author's individual journey and viewpoints on weight loss.

The medical information presented in this book is not intended as professional advice and should not be regarded as such. It is crucial not to replace the guidance of qualified physicians with this information. The content is of a general nature and is intended to enhance readers' awareness of their healthcare. It is always advisable to seek personalized guidance from your medical practitioner to address your specific requirements. For concerns pertaining to your health and any symptoms that may necessitate diagnosis or medical intervention, it is recommended to consult a medical professional.

DEDICATION

Dedicated to all those who tried to lose weight, were disappointed in the results and lost faith in the possibility of this matter. I myself passed through this whole painful path, which seemed to be a vicious circle, but I was able to find a way out of it and I know for sure that you will succeed too, do not lose hope and go for it!

CONTENTS

ACKNOWLEDGMENTS

I want to thank God and the Saints who guide me.
I want to thank my husband, my children and my parents for support.

1. HOW TO USE AGILE TO LOSE WEIGHT

What's "Agile?" The term "Agile" comes from the IT (Information Technologies) field. It denotes a specific methodology of conducting software development projects. The Agile approach has shown its effectiveness in IT, and now Agile is penetrating into various other areas of our everyday and professional lives, becoming widespread in companies from various industries.

Agile means taking an iterative approach to solving a task. One part of a large task is solved within a specific period of time (iteration). Planning is carried out at the beginning of each iteration, and a discussion is held at the end of the iteration about which results were achieved. The Agile approach requires a lot of communication, and the customer is deeply involved in the process of coming up with a solution. After all, it is up to the customer to decide whether they have received a complete solution to their original task or not.

As a result, Agile helps reduce the possibility of receiving something but the product they were looking for once the development is finished. Here is a classic example from the IT field:

You have an idea for a mobile application. You have come up with what to do, and how to do it. You have found developers, and explained everything to them, and they nodded that they understood it all. They said they would get the whole job done in 3 months, and that suited you, so went you home to wait. Let us say 4 months later, you look at the completed project, and you do not see anything even slightly resembling what you wanted to do! Time passed, and you have not gotten any results. Why is this happening? There could be many reasons: you did not check to make sure that the IT team understood your story correctly to begin with;

your idea changed over the last 4 months and the developers did not know that; or our fast world has changed again, and your original idea lost its relevance...

Agile approach suggests splitting such a project into small, short cycles, called iterations (also called sprints). These are periods during that a certain cycle of actions is performed to fulfill part of your project. Agile mandates showing the customer the results obtained, followed by a discussion about how this or that turned out. This discussion goes hand in hand with adjustments to ideas, plans, and tasks for the next iteration. This creates greater involvement in the process of working on the project, facilitates control of the work carried out, and makes it possible to make on the go. Planning for the next sprint takes the data analyzed at the end of the current sprint into account. Some work is added, while other tasks are removed from the plan as being irrelevant. As a customer or developer, you always know what state your project is in, and what you can expect from it in the near future. Each iteration is in fact a separate project, and ideally, you have a ready-made version of some part of your product at the end of each iteration. Another feature of Agile methodologies is reducing the amount of written documentation that describes the project. Is that a good thing? It sure is! Therefore, it is no surprise that not only IT specialists use this approach.

In general, it is fascinating to observe how people implement the principles of flexible project management in other fields. In the IT company where I work, Agile principles are applied not only when working on specific IT projects, but also to other non-core areas, such as the process of recruitment and work with personnel, PR and marketing, and other team activities, like organizing large conferences.

I am friends with several people who use Agile approach in their family, and in parenting. This includes weekly family meetings with discussions on plans and ideas for the near future, as well as process of setting tasks for the iteration for each family member, depending on their ability to fulfill them. Monitoring the tasks, performed by children and other family members, helps to instill responsibility, and make everyone feel like a united family team.

So, is it possible apply principles of Agile methodology for such tasks as: losing weight, changing yourself, your diet and your lifestyle, adding physical activities to your daily routine, embedding all this into your real life. Of course! Moreover, you should! So how?

With the Agile approach, you will not have a single diet option that you have to adhere to at all costs, though you may already "hate" the diet for what it makes you do. In contrast to traditional approach on losing weight, there will not be neither one universal set of exercises that supposedly suits everyone equally, nor generally accepted rules, like "don't eat after 6:00 p.m." You have already tried these things, and you did not get any results. Only despair.

I suggest that you consider losing weight in the Agile style as a process of creating your own unique lifestyle. You analyze your own life situation and the state of your body, taking into account your own emotional and psychological state at a particular time, knowing your body's features and quirks. Then, using collected data, you can develop your own, individual, system of weight loss, adjusting nutrition and physical activity. It can be affected by numerous parameters, such as: your weight, age, level of physical activity, love or dislike for specific foods and methods of preparation, types of training (gym, walking, etc.), meal schedule, sleep and wakefulness rhythm, work schedule, mother-in-law's visits on Saturdays, trips to the countryside for fresh air, and other factors that are important to you personally. You can carefully analyze all this and develop an individual weight loss plan for the first sprint — the one that you are ready to fulfill, while also having fun. Then you can follow your plan for a while, be it a week, or two, or a month. This is your personal sprint. After that, you analyze your results. What have you achieved? What has not worked yet? What did you wish you could stop doing? Something that did not fit, something you did not like, some elements of your plan that you want to replace. Then, based on these new data, you make adjustments and get a new weight loss plan for your next sprint.

In our rapidly changing world, sticking to an "unshakable" diet and a stable training schedule can be very challenging. Your work and lifestyle may interfere with your weight loss plans. Sudden business trips, interesting vacations, closure of gyms, self-isolation in an apartment, lack of certain ingredients necessary for your specific diet, and other external factors can affect your ability to follow your diet and training regime. The Agile approach to weight loss assumes that state of your body and mind, environment at work and home, your day-to-day routine are always changing. This input data cannot be constant, so you have to adjust. You need to take these changes into account when planning your schedule for the next sprint (by the way, the current sprint can also be revised, but only if a sudden situation occurs that changes your life, as, for example, happened with COVID). Consider incoming problems as they arise, and solve them in the simplest and fastest way possible.

2. ADOPTING AGILE MANIFESTO FOR WEIGHT LOSE PROJECT

Agile manifesto, which was declared by software engineers in US in 2001, has its own set of values:
- individuals and interactions over processes and tools;
- working software over comprehensive documentation;
- customer collaboration over contract negotiation;
- responding to change over following a plan.

The full text of the Agile manifesto can be found here https://agilemanifesto.org/iso/en/manifesto.html.

If we rephrase these ideas of the Agile manifesto using the context of weight loss, they may sound as follows:

- Your health, both physical and psychological, is more important than your desire to lose weight, and the methods and tools used for weight loss (your health is more important than what nutritionists and fitness instructors tell you to do).

- If you've chosen a weight loss approach that works for you, and you lose kilograms, but you don't have time to write down the "recipe" for your weight loss in a notebook — that's fine.

- Listening to yourself, understanding your body, and staying in harmony with yourself is much more important than the numbers your scale show. Cooperation with yourself as a customer, taking into account your lifestyle, family, work, food and sports preferences, and other conditions, is more important than relentlessly following an unshakable plan solely based on your desire to lose a certain number of kilograms.

- Responding to changes is more important than following the original plan (this point is unchanged).

3. PLANNING TO LOSE WEGHT WITH AGILE APPROACH

I decided to try the Agile approach and tools intuitively after yet another unsuccessful attempt to push myself through a newfangled diet. I tried changing my approach, using the methodology of conducting IT projects as a basis for my weight loss project. After all, they get results, despite the constant changes and limitations of technology and hardware. I was confident — this methodology would work in my project, even though it was a weight loss project.

So, what do you need to take into account, what do you need to foresee, and what are you able to do, to implement Agile in your own weight loss program?

1. Collect initial data.

The first thing to do is to measure and record your initial data. Measure everything that can be measured: your weight, clothing size, body measurements (bust, waist, hips, etc.) and, for example, remember which hole you use to fasten your belt. Calculate everything that can be — your body mass index, waist-hip index, etc.

Now you need to record all this data. Write it in a diary and/or save it in a digital format (on laptop, smartphone) indicating the date when you made the measurements.

It is good to see your progress so, I suggest you take pictures of your body from different angles (from the front, sides and back).

2. Choose your planning interval.

It's time to decide for how long you're ready to plan your iteration, be it a month, a week, or two weeks. This will be your Sprint. The main thing that you commit to is to follow all the plans and "rules" that you outline for yourself throughout the Sprint. Of course, some of your ideas related to nutrition and physical activity may fall out. For example, due to allergies to a certain food, or coming down with a cold. In general, you need to make your initial plan simple enough for you to accomplish in this Sprint.

3. Set a goal, outline a plan and act.

The next step is to decide on the nearest realistic goal, and outline steps to achieve it. Write down a specific goal in your diary and an estimated plan of how you expect to act. Structure your plan block by block: nutrition, physical activity, habits. Specify which foods you will eat, how you will cook them, in what quantity (in ounces or grams), how often you will eat, what kind of physical activity you plan to do, and in what amount, and what you are thinking of giving up. Your plan should not be abstract. "I give my word of honor that I will do exercises and eat right" — that would not do. Instead, write down a specific menu and a physical training schedule in a notebook. Perfect plan is the one that fits into your lifestyle. It must go together with your work, your household chores, and other routine tasks. Menu for each day should take into account what kind of food you take with you to work. It should also include information about exercises, when and what kind of physical activity you do. "I exercise at home for 45 minutes watching my favorite TV show that starts at 9 p.m. In addition to that, I get off the bus one stop earlier than usual to walk the rest of the way." The more specific and detailed your plan is, the better!

Now when the plan is ready, you start living according to our approved schedule, taking no detours throughout our sprint. During this process, you take notes of everything that does not work for us, and you notice features and details that become clearer as you move towards our goal. Then you come up with new tasks that you think will help us reduce weight, and you write them all down in our diary. This will help you understand what is happening to your body, how it reacts to new nutrition and new activities. Also, record in your diary all the features related to the state of your health, well-being, and feelings: successes and failures, what is working and what is not, breakdowns, etc.

4. Analyze results.

At the end of the iteration, it is time to sum up the interim results and analyze the results according to the parameters you measured at the beginning: weigh yourself at about the same time on the same scales, measure yourself with the same measuring tape, try to button the same clothes, and take photos from all the same angles as before. All this data will be useful for our analysis.

Compare your results, scroll through your diary, and summarize the results. Have you gotten closer to your goal? Are you moving in the right direction?

5.   Start the next Sprint.

In the next iteration, you should take only what worked well in the last sprint: what you liked, what turned out well, and what you would like to repeat. You should not include anything in the new iteration that was useless or did not take root. Think of new ingredients that can replace the foods that seemed tasteless. Think of what can replace exercises that you found uninteresting or difficult. Analyze whether it is possible to change something else in your lifestyle to fit your new system of nutrition and training. Do you have some new ideas on how to diversify your menu, or minimize your time spent cooking? Do you have enough energy to increase your level of daily physical activity without "harming" your work, family, or business? Analyze the mistakes and plan everything to avoid these mistakes in the new iteration.

The results you obtain, and the results that you evaluated at the end of the first iteration, now become new input data for the next period, for the next sprint. Now the cycle repeats from the beginning, acting in iterations, comparing our appearance, our well-being, and our mood, as well as all the digital indicators that you control, gradually moving towards your goal.

4. BORROWING AGILE TOOLS

There are different ways (frameworks) within an Agile approach to organize the processes of project management and quality control. Among the most popular of them in IT are Scrum and Kanban. Both of these frameworks have a lot of features and tools designed to help developers cope with the difficulties of working on a project that has unclear requirements. These systems can be very useful for your weight loss project.

Backlog — a list of wishes and tasks for the entire project

Think of all your wishes, possible tasks, and important steps that are related to weight loss process. Write them all down in a single list. Add any tasks you like or ideas you want to try once you get the opportunity, but cannot at this moment. You should also add new tasks to the backlog as your work on the project progresses as you discover new things. At the beginning of each sprint, you will take a bunch of tasks for your planned iteration from this list.

Daily Scrum Meetings

In IT projects, all project participants meet up for a daily meeting. This allows synchronizing the team members, so that everyone understands the general context and the statuses of the tasks performed. Everyone exchanges information by answering three standard questions:

- What did I do yesterday that helped me get closer to the sprint goal?
- What will I do today to help achieve the sprint goal?

- Do I see any obstacles that might prevent me from reaching the sprint goal?

In your case, this means conducting a regular analysis of your progress on task list. You ask yourself the same three questions at a "meeting" with yourself.

Scrum or Kanban Board

In IT projects, whiteboards are often used as a tool for visualizing the status of project tasks and the project as a whole. Visually representation shows the percentage of completion, how much the team is using its potential, what the existing problems and difficulties are, etc. Physically, these can be marker boards, or cork boards with sticky notes, or software (computer) implementations, such as the Trello tool. It can even mean just drawing tables with tasks in a diary, and so on.

Both Scrum and Kanban are varieties of flexible approaches based on different principles. Scrum relies on the chosen pace of your work — the goal here is to complete the whole sprint on time. In contrast, Kanban's focus is on task lists, and the goal is to complete the task on time.

Kanban was born at Toyota as a lean manufacturing system, and the word itself translates as "signal card." Kanban has the greatest flexibility — using this method you can add tasks at any time, or postpone the end of the sprint to another day for good reasons.

Your weight loss is a "solo" project: you are the customer, the performer of the work tasks, and the evaluator of goal achievement. You will integrate the process into real life, and you will need maximum flexibility.

Kanban Card

Main component of Kanban is a card — a visual element that shows the particular task on the board. For example, one of the biggest tasks that you cannot skip when losing weight is restricting your diet, eating a healthy, balanced diet.

If you write, "Eat a healthy, balanced diet" on a card on the board, I doubt that you will be able to successfully complete this task and transfer it right away to the completed column.

It would be logical to divide the task "Eat a healthy, balanced diet" into the following small tasks:

- learn the basics of nutrition physiology;
- calculate the amount of nutrients and calories at which you'll still be able to lose weight;

- learn the basics of healthy diet, proper nutrition, buy a corresponding book;
- decide on a menu for the upcoming week;
- buy groceries for the week ahead;
- search for recipes and information about how to cook delicious dishes from the groceries you've chosen;
- write down your menu for the day.

For various people the task of "Eat a healthy, balanced diet" can be divided into a number of various small subtasks that they will write on Kanban cards.

Of course, your Kanban weight loss board is just a tool for you to use. The success of the entire project, i.e. achievement of your desired result, will mostly depend on your motivation, discipline and the knowledge that you possess.

5. "SLENDERNESS BOARD"

So, have you decided to use agile methodologies and tools for your weight loss project? Now you have a general idea of the principles and approaches, but how exactly should you start your weight loss project?

Let us go step-by-step.

1. **Define your weight-loss goal.**

How many pounds or kilograms are you planning to lose? Be realistic.

2. **Define the starting and completion dates.**

Based on your weight-loss goal and considering your body's real possibilities, determine when you are ready to start and for how long you are committed to achieve desirable results.

Since you are embedding your weight loss project into your existing lifestyle, without planning to quit your job, family, and loved ones, and move to a desert island, I suggest choosing the most convenient day for you to start your project. Use the same day of the week in the future for you to start new Sprint after summing up the results of current one. On this day you should dedicate enough time for a "meeting" with yourself. If it is difficult to choose among working days, probably you need a one day off – starting may be difficult, but as process started, it would be easy to support it. Let us say you chose Monday, after you have sent your children to school and your husband to work, you can allocate time to coordinate your "slimming" project. This time you need to analyze results of previous Sprint and set up a plan for next coming Sprint.

In my experience, it would be important to choose a starting date when you are situated in your usual circumstances, under the same conditions in which you typically spend most of your time. If you know you are going on a business trip or vacation in the near future, think to yourself — is it worth starting your project right now? Is it possible you will get bad results because external circumstances outweigh your new "beginnings" with an unusual nutrition and training schedule? It is difficult for someone else to decide for you whether you will be able to resist the temptations that you will encounter on the way. On the other hand, there is no sense waiting and postponing the start of your weight loss. There will never be better conditions than right now. The desire to "postpone something for later" is a psychological trick that causes you to never start a new lifestyle altogether. You do want to lose weight, am I right? Can you start right now? Go ahead and get to work!

3.   Determine the duration of your Sprints.

The shorter Sprint the more often you review results and reconsider plans. I would recommend using weekly iterations. For example, by summing up the results on Saturday after the workweek, you can relax a little in the evening of this day and give yourself a cheat meal. You can also use biweekly or monthly sprints to eliminate weekly fluctuations with numbers you can get because of different factors can affect weekly results (menstrual cycle, carbohydrate intake, swelling, colds, intense workouts, etc.).

6. ORGANIZE YOUR "SLENDERNESS BOARD"

This can be a marker board, corkboard, paperboard that hangs on the wall, a page of your diary, or a specialized app on your phone.

The main idea of working with your "Slenderness Board" is that writing tasks on stickers, gluing stickers or moving cards in electronic version of your board helps you visualize your progress. You can observe all tasks and their statuses, so you will not forget to execute everything.

The table should contain a set of columns.

- **The column "BACKLOG / ALL TASKS AND WISHES"**

This is a general list of tasks/wishes/proposed solutions/ideas that will help you lose weight. Therefore, it contains all the tasks that you feel are important for you to perform during your entire weight loss project. Examples include: to get examined by your doctor; to study proper nutrition systems (a healthy food, balanced diet); to calculate your ideal body weight and daily metabolism; to watch a video each day on how to lose weight; to listen to podcasts about proper nutrition on the way to work; to start running; to do sit-ups and light exercises while watching TV in the evening; to drink 2 liters of water a day; to normalize your sleep; to start taking multivitamins; to buy membership in a gym or a professional swimming pool; to buy a mat and dumbbells for sports; to give up sugar in coffee; to buy a sugar replacement, etc.

All new tasks that will arise in the course of your weight loss journey go to this column. From this column you will select tasks for each new sprint.

How to formulate your tasks depends entirely on you. A lot may depend on the wording. For example, "looking for a gym" and "going to training on Tuesdays and Thursdays" can look like very different tasks. If "looking for a gym" really leads you to go for trainings – good for you, but if you need detailed calls to actions – split the task to "find a gym to subscribe by next Friday" and "go training each Monday and Friday at 6 p.m." Do as suits for you, the main thing is that you get closer to your goal.

At the beginning of each new Sprint, your board has to have next clear mandatory three columns.

- **The column "TO DO"**

Here you put those activities that you plan to perform in the current sprint, take the most relevant tasks from the backlog, and only as many as you think you will actually have time to complete in this iteration.

For each sprint, try to choose tasks from various areas, such as restrict your diet and get more physical activity, check your health status and visit a doctor, change your lifestyle and give up certain bad habits, etc. Choosing many different tasks from the same area for one sprint may not be the most effective solution. If you choose only physical activities, like doing exercises at home, going to the gym 3 times a week, running 5 km every morning, and going to the pool twice a week — it may be unrealistic to do all this. Moreover, it may not provide your expected effect within a comprehensive solution to the multifactorial problem of excess weight.

- **The column "IN PROGRESS"**

Put your tasks that are currently in progress here. This, on the one hand, will serve as a reminder of what needs to be done today, while on the other hand helping you concentrate on analyzing each task that needs to be carried out daily. Choose a time that is convenient for you, in the morning over a cup of coffee, or in the evening in silence, or at lunchtime, alone with your diary. See what you have been able to do, what you forgot, and what obstacles you have encountered on the way to fulfilling specific tasks. For example, if the pool is closed for cleaning, you need to either look for a different, suitable pool, or postpone the "Go to the pool" card until another sprint, when the pool finally re-opens.

- **The column "DONE"**

To this column, you place all completed tasks. Some tasks upon completion can allow starting another task. For example, if the "Buy multivitamins" task is done, then you can move the "Take multivitamins daily" card to the

"IN PROGRESS" column. This task will remind you about multivitamins during all the sprint duration. If you do not need reminders – you may not use a card for reminding and vice versa – you may need many reminding cards in case you have many different nutritional supplements to take, you can add dosage and scheme of taking to corresponding reminding cards. This is your board, so make it work for you in a best way.

At the end of each Sprint, conduct a retrospective analysis of what you accomplished, what you failed, and for what reasons.

At the beginning of each Sprint, you should update your board with new tasks chosen from the backlog list or transferred (in case of recurrent tasks, for example) from current board, according to your plan for the coming Sprint.

7 YOUR BOARD, YOUR RULES

How to customize your board.

Above we described mandatory columns for your board, but you can name and organize the columns in a way convenient for you, and correlates meaningfully with your lifestyle.

- **"DAILY TASKS"**

For example, you can add this column where you will place all your tasks that remain with you constantly. Such tasks as "Do daily light exercises at home," "Drink 2 liters of water daily," "Take vitamins daily" suits well to this column.

- **"I'M DONE!"**

You can use such a column to keep your achievements you are proud of here. This column will grow, delight and motivate you.

- **"MISTAKES"**

This column is for those actions that regularly lead to mistakes that prevent you from moving towards your weight loss goal. For example, "I didn't go to bed on time," "I ate too much," "I got the munchies before my menstruation" or "Breakdowns during stress," "Taking irregular meals" and so on. Knowing factors that counterbalance your efforts to lose weight, you will be able to arm yourself with a means of confrontation. Organizing a supply of useful "goodies"; setting an alarm clock with a lullaby as a reminder of sleeping time; taking the right snacks with you if it is impossible to organize a full lunch, etc.

- **"BLACK SWAN"**

If you encounter sudden circumstances that interfere with your sprint, make sure you add that to your board too. For example, getting a cold can force you to adjust the weight loss process, and you will need to reduce your physical activity, review your nutrition, add vitamins, stay at home and cancel scheduled visits to gyms, massages and so on. All of this should be taken into account in your "Slenderness Board."

What else could be customized?

You can use markers or stickers of different colors, add labels in the application (in Trello) to indicate different task categories (nutrition, fitness, motivation, general, lifestyle, etc.). Visually "multicoloration" of cards/tasks in the current iteration will clearly show that you are working on your weight loss project in a balanced way from different angles.

Be creative – add any customizations you want. Your board helps you to maintain your information dominance, which is the main factor for motivation to lose weight. Every day, looking at and analyzing you board, you are getting deeply focused on your losing weight project.

Do not forget that the board is just a tool for working on your project. If you are not achieving your desired results, there may be something wrong with the approaches you have chosen. Remember that finding a working for you scheme for weight loss is more important than board itself.

Responding to change is more important than following your original plan. Analyze more what you are doing and what worked and what not for you and adopt your plans accordingly.

Tools are here to support you, choose any form you like. Have you tried using the electronic version of your "Slenderness Board" and realized that it does not suit you? Do social networks suck you in when you open a board on your phone? Try other options, draw columns on a large poster on the wall of the refrigerator, and stick colorful stickers on it with your tasks. This way your board will be in a prominent place, and at moments of weakness, when you want to steal some forbidden yummy treat from the refrigerator, your board will help you resist your impulsive desires.

8. TASK

So, are you ready to try using Agile methodology tools to lose weight right now? Have you decided where you will keep your board? Will it be a marker board or a corkboard on the wall, an online app. or two pages in your diary? Take action!

1. Hold a meeting with yourself and formulate goals, then set deadlines, your Sprint duration, etc.
2. Following the results of the "meeting," record a backlog with tasks for your entire project.
3. Draw your board with selected columns (remember that we need three main columns for the sprint, a list of all tasks, and the remaining columns if desired).
4. In the columns "TO DO" and "IN PROGRESS" write out your specific plans for completing tasks for the current sprint. If you have already completed something from the plans outlined in your head, indicate that in the column "DONE." Be sure to praise yourself by signing: "Well done! Keep it up!"
5. Now everything is ready! Just glance at your board every day, or open an online app with your board, and hold a meeting with yourself. What are you planning to do today from the list of tasks in the corresponding column? What are you already doing? What tasks are you working on this week? What has already been done? Drag the task lines between the columns, re-stick your stickers, or rewrite the tasks in your diary.
6. Do not forget to take the peculiarities of your lifestyle, work schedule and sudden events into account. All this should be reflected in the board every day if it affects how you lose weight.

7. At the end of the sprint, you need to allocate more time than usual for summing up, performing a retrospective analysis of what you got done during the iteration, and what you failed to do. What were the reasons for why you did not manage to implement one of the planned tasks? Did you take on too much off the bat for this sprint? Did you fail to calculate your endurance properly? Did unexpected external factors interfere, or is something wrong with your management of your board? Analyze your sprint results: have you achieved some intermediate goal in losing weight? Praise yourself even for small achievements! Did you stick to your diet plan almost perfectly during the sprint? Did you miss one training session for a very good reason? Instead, you took a walk in the park with an old friend — a great alternative. Were you motivated every day of the last sprint? Well done! Sweet! Now keep moving on. Write down your errors in a separate column, in order to try to avoid them by all known legal means.

8. We are planning tasks for the next Sprint, taking the conclusions made from the previous one into account. Collect as many tasks from the backlog, as you are able to complete, and exactly those that are relevant in this iteration. And that's it, voila! Let us move on to a new sprint of your weight loss using flexible Agile methodologies.

9. Enjoy the results you've achieved!

9. MY EXPERIENCE OF FINDING A FLEXIBLE WAY

I, like many people, started losing weight with fashionable diets and exercise complexes, but, not getting the desired results, fortunately, I did not just abandon this idea of losing weight, but looked for other approaches, so my Agile path was formed.

At the beginning of my weight program, it was difficult for me to give up the usual sweet and fatty foods, such as chocolate, honey, butter, dried fruits, etc. I could not refuse, but I limited their number so that the kilograms would go away. However, at some point the scales stopped showing a decrease. I realized then that even small amounts of my favorite foods from fast carbohydrates and fats add enough energy value that without this, I would have a big enough calorie deficit to lose weight. You can gradually reduce foods that interfere with your weight loss, and replace them with other foods or cooking methods that will give you weight loss results. You will not need to switch abruptly from your usual diet to "no food at all" or to "cabbage only," which will inevitably provoke a terrible breakdown and, as a result, the return of lost kilograms (or even a weight gain). You do not need to become another victim of a low-calorie and unbalanced diet and gain even more weight, instead of losing weight.

For example, I love the traditional recipe for cheesecake (farmer's cheese, eggs, flour, sugar, and jam on top), but over time I have adapted my recipe to fit my requirements. Ordinary cottage cheese is replaced with low-fat, sugar with a sweetener, whole eggs with egg whites, the amount of flour can either be significantly reduced or a small amount of rice / almond / buckwheat or oatmeal ground in a coffee grinder can be used instead of wheat flour, jam is successfully replaced with fresh or freshly frozen berries. This cheesecake turns out to be a delicious, lower-calorie dish that may well find a place in your "losing weight" diet. If you build up a small calorie deficit during the day, you will lose weight even when eating dishes like this.

I took just as flexible an approach with carbohydrates. At the beginning, my menu was quite extensive. I ate porridges of various kinds, legumes, and starchy vegetables (pumpkin, potatoes, carrots, and beets). As I lost weight, I realized that even a small amount of potatoes or baked pumpkin affected the results I saw on the scales at the end of the sprint. I have introduced myself new porridges, adding and removing ingredients, monitoring my overall feeling, my sense of being full, and the weight loss results I am achieving.

As soon as you realize that your diet and physical activity in this iteration are not helping you to get results, then stop and analyze what exactly is not working, and what should be changed. It is possible that the matter is not in the products themselves, but in their quantity, or method of preparation. For example, "dietary" farmer's cheese pancakes, despite all their nutritional value, can have a negative effect on weight loss when eaten in large quantities, since they are fried in oil. If you do not understand what exactly in your diet is preventing you from losing weight, you can try to change your ingredients completely in the next iteration. For example, if you have had a lot of beef and fatty fish on the menu, try changing it to turkey and low-fat white fish. Try various experiments, but be sure to record your results, in order to understand what suits you and what does not.

Use the same approach with regard to physical activity. If you do not see any result from aerobics classes in a group, from classes with a certain coach in a particular gym, when you freeze in the pool or "suffer" in yoga, then do not force yourself to continue. We can afford to do what we like, and avoid unpleasant things, especially aiming to our health. This, of course, does not mean you can just not do anything if you do not like it. Find and select such a training schedule and such types of physical activity that will suit you and will give results at the end of the next iteration.

What about your personal experience?

1. Remember your previous attempts to lose weight. Which of the foods you ate do you think contributed to weight loss at that time? Are you ready to try including them again in your diet? What parts of your diet are preventing you from losing weight? What can you replace these products with, or how can you change your recipe and cooking method?
2. It is the same with physical activity. Which gym did you visit? Did you

like it, and do you want to go back? Which exercises were successful and gave you results?

3. Have you drawn up your board? Have you thought through your sprints? Have you made a list of the tasks that you will start with?

4. Make sure that you have figured out how to integrate a new schedule of meals and physical activity into your usual life schedule. Have holidays, business trips, New Year's, birthdays and other important dates been taken into account?

5. Have you already written everything down in your weight loss diary? Then go for it!

10. BE FLEXIBLE

Believe in yourself and you will succeed.

The most important thing you have already done — you have realized that you need to be slim to maintain your health, so then just follow your goal. Do not give up, even if something does not work right away, just change approaches, methods, ways, be flexible. Losing weight is a long process, because you have been gaining excess weight for years and physiologically impossible to get rid of it in a couple of weeks. You need to look at weight loss as a big project with different length phases and intermediate metrics.

I devoted a lot of time studying how energy metabolism works in cells, how to effectively use nutrition and physical activity to reduce excess weight without harming the body. My experience and knowledge is described in a large book that became the source of this series of books, the first of which you are now holding in your hands. I know for sure that before your scales show the desired figure, it will be necessary to thank your body many times for small but very important changes.

Working in the IT sphere, I was acquainted with modern Agile project management methodologies, with their handy planning and controlling tools that will help you remember the main things and build your individual weight loss system. This is a project you can manage flexibly, pause, travel, give yourself a break from dieting and come back with a new menu and a new workout schedule.

Health is our top priority. The series of this book is about taking a conscious approach to your body and getting yourself in the shape that will help you feel good and be happy with yourself.

I wish you to make your dreams come true!

27

ABOUT THE AUTHOR

Elena Fedorova holds a degree in Medicine (Neurologist) and has additional education in Fitness Training and Nutrition. With 18 years of experience in the field of Information Technology, she has worked with modern software development methodologies at one global software development company. Elena has also established and coordinated various IT communities, for technological experts and newbies, for women in IT, for tech leaders who want to mentor in the IT industry, etc. She writes articles, gives interviews, and speaks at events on IT project management, personnel management, and motivation.

Combining her medical background, experience in IT project management methodologies, and a passion for weight loss and healthy living, Elena has developed her own weight loss methodology. Several years ago, she successfully lost 30 kg herself using this approach, which has also helped many others struggling with weight loss. Elena frequently receives feedback about how she inspires people to take action and make positive changes. Her goal is to inspire as many individuals as possible who wish to achieve a healthy weight and provide them with an easy-to-follow methodology to accomplish their goals.

If you have any questions, comments, ideas please do not hesitate to contact me via email fedorovaalena.com@gmail.com.

You can find more information on book's page
https://www.facebook.com/agilehealthbook
https://www.instagram.com/fedorovaalena/